# Understanding cancer of the pancreas

This booklet is for you if you have or someone close to you has cancer of the pancreas and you want to know more about its treatment.

It has been prepared and checked by cancer doctors, other relevant specialists, nurses and patients. Together they represent an agreed view on this cancer, its diagnosis and management, and the key aspects of living with it.

If you are a patient your doctor or nurse may wish to go through the booklet with you and mark sections that are particularly important for you. You can make a note below of the main contacts and information that you may need quickly.

**Specialist nurse/contact names**

. . . . . . . . . . . . . . . . . . . . . . . . . . . . .

. . . . . . . . . . . . . . . . . . . . . . . . . . . . .

**Hospital**

**Phone** . . . . . . . . . . . . . . . . . . . . . . . .

**Treatments** . . . . . . . . . . . . . . . . . . .

. . . . . . . . . . . . . . . . . . . . . . . . . . . . .

. . . . . . . . . . . . . . . . . . . . . . . . . . . . .

**Family doctor**

. . . . . . . . . . . . . . . . . . . . . . . . . . . . .

. . . . . . . . . . . . . . . . . . . . . . . . . . . . .

**Surgery address**

*If you like you can also add:*

**Your name** . . . . . . . . . . . . . . . . . . . .

**Address**. . . . . . . . . . . . . . . . . . . . . . .

. . . . . . . . . . . . . . . . . . . . . . . . . . . . .

# Understanding cancer of the pancreas – key points in this booklet

This booklet aims to tell you about cancer of the pancreas, how it is diagnosed and treated and how the treatment may affect you.

These two pages sum up the main points, and show which pages to turn to for more information.

### What causes cancer of the pancreas? Page 9

Very little is known about the causes of cancer of the pancreas, but there is a slightly greater risk in people who smoke.

### What are the symptoms of cancer of the pancreas? Page 10

The symptoms may include:
- yellowing of the skin and whites of the eyes }
- dark yellow urine                             } jaundice
- pale bowel motions                           }
- loss of appetite and weight
- pain in the upper abdomen and back

**Obviously, most pain in the abdomen is not caused by cancer of the pancreas, but see your doctor if you are worried.**

### How is cancer of the pancreas diagnosed? Pages 11-14

Various tests are used, including:

- ultrasound scan
- CT scan
- MRI scan
- ERCP test
- biopsy

## What types of treatment are used? Pages 14-15

Surgery is the main treatment if the cancer can be completely removed. Radiotherapy, often combined with chemotherapy, can be used to treat cancers that cannot be removed by surgery, but which have not spread beyond the pancreas. Chemotherapy may be used to treat cancers that have spread.

## How will I feel during and after treatment? Pages 25-30

You may feel anxious, afraid or angry because of the cancer, the treatment and its effects.

The worst fear is often fear of the unknown.

It may help you to find out as much as you can about the cancer, its treatment, and living with it.

Do not be afraid to ask, and go on asking until you get the information and support you need.

## For more information

Many people and organisations can help. This booklet lists useful organisations (pages 38-40), books that might help (pages 41-42), and BACUP's booklets (page 43).

The nurses in BACUP's cancer information service (0171 613 2121 or Freephone 0800 18 11 99) can give information about all aspects of cancer, and people who can help.

If you need to talk through your feelings in depth, you can contact BACUP's cancer counselling service on 0171 696 9000, or at BACUP Scotland in Glasgow on 0141 553 1553.

3 Bath Place, Rivington Street, London, EC2A 3JR

BACUP was founded by Dr Vicky Clement-Jones, following her own experiences with ovarian cancer, and offers information, counselling and support to people with cancer, their families and friends.

We produce publications on the main types of cancer, treatments, and ways of living with cancer. We also produce a magazine, *BACUP News,* three times a year.

Our success depends on feedback from users of the service. We thank everyone, particularly patients and their families, whose advice has made this booklet possible.

Administration 0171 696 9003
Cancer Support Service:
Information 0171 613 2121 (8 lines) or Freeline 0800 18 11 99
Counselling 0171 696 9000 (London)
BACUP Scotland Cancer Counselling Service
0141 553 1553 (Glasgow)

British Association of Cancer United Patients and their families and friends.
A company limited by guarantee. Registered in England and Wales
company number 2803321. Charity registration number 1019719.
Registered office 3 Bath Place, Rivington Street, London, EC2A 3JR

*Medical consultant: Dr Maurice Slevin, MD, FRCP*

*Editor: Stella Wood*

*Illustrations: Andrew Macdonald & Peter Gardiner*

*Cover design: Alison Hooper Associates*

First published 1993, reprinted 1995, revised 1997

Typeset and printed in Great Britain by Lithoflow Ltd., London

ISBN 1-870403-99-1

# Contents

# Introduction

This booklet has been written to help you understand more about cancer of the pancreas. We hope it answers some of the questions you may have about its diagnosis and treatment, and addresses some of the feelings which are a large part of anyone's reaction to a cancer diagnosis.

We can't advise you about the best treatment for yourself because this information can only come from your own doctor, who will be familiar with your full medical history.

At the end of this booklet you will find a list of other BACUP publications, some useful addresses and recommended books, and a page to fill in with any questions you may have for your doctor or nurse. If, after reading this booklet, you think it has helped you, do pass it on to any of your family and friends who might find it interesting. They too may want to be informed so they can help you cope with any problems you may have.

# What is cancer?

The organs and tissues of the body are made up of tiny building blocks called cells. Cancer is a disease of these cells. Although cells in different parts of the body may look and work differently, most repair and reproduce themselves in the same way. Normally, this division of cells takes place in an orderly and controlled manner. If, for some reason, the process gets out of control, the cells will continue to divide, developing into a lump which is called a **tumour**. Tumours can be either **benign** or **malignant**.

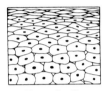 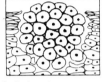

Normal cells      Cells forming a tumour

In a benign tumour the cells do not spread to other parts of the body and so are not cancerous. If they continue to grow at the original site, however, they may cause a problem by pressing on the surrounding organs.

A malignant tumour consists of cancer cells which have the ability to spread beyond the original site. If the tumour is left untreated, it may invade and destroy surrounding tissue. Sometimes cells break away from the original (**primary**) cancer and spread to other organs in the body via the bloodstream or lymphatic system. When these cells reach a new site they may go on dividing and form a new tumour, often referred to as a **secondary** or a **metastasis**.

Doctors can tell whether a tumour is benign or malignant by examining a small sample of cells under a microscope. This is called a **biopsy.**

It is important to realise that cancer is not a single disease with a single cause and a single type of treatment. There are more than 200 different kinds of cancer, each with its own name and treatment.

# The pancreas

The pancreas is a gland that lies in the upper half of the abdomen, well above the umbilicus, at the V where the ribs meet in front. It is about six inches long. The large rounded section on the right-hand side of the body is called the head of the pancreas, the mid-section is known as the body of the pancreas and the narrow part on the left-hand side of the body is called the tail of the pancreas. The head of the pancreas lies next to the first part of the small intestine called the duodenum.

The pancreas secretes pancreatic juice – a fluid which helps with the process of digestion – and insulin – a hormone which enables the body to use sugars and store fats.

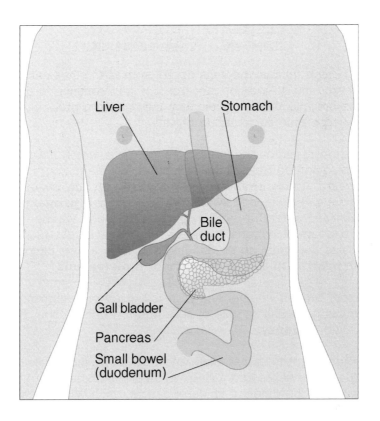

# What causes cancer of the pancreas?

Very little is known about the causes of pancreatic cancer but there is a slightly greater risk in people who smoke cigarettes.

A condition called chronic pancreatitis, where the pancreas becomes inflamed, is a possible cause in a minority of cases.

Cancer of the pancreas is slightly more common in men than in women. It arises mainly in older people and is rare below the age of 50.

# What are the different types of cancer of the pancreas?

Most cancer of the pancreas arises from the cells on the inner lining of the ducts – the channels through which the fluids produced by the pancreas flow out. It occurs more frequently in the head of the pancreas than in the body or the tail.

The other type of pancreatic cancer is extremely rare and is a tumour of the cells that produce insulin. This is known as islet cell cancer.

# What are the symptoms of cancer of the pancreas?

If the cancer develops in the head of the pancreas then it may block the bile duct which carries the bile from the liver to the intestine. This causes the bile to be retained in the body and results in the skin and whites of the eyes becoming yellow; the urine also becomes a dark yellow colour, and stools (bowel motions) are pale. This is known as jaundice.

Other symptoms of cancer of the pancreas are usually vague and non-specific. The cancer may not cause any symptoms for a long time. You may feel discomfort or pain in the upper abdomen which sometimes spreads to the back. In the beginning the pain may come and go but later on it is more persistent. In some people the pain is worse while lying down and it is relieved by sitting up or bending forward. You may also have been losing weight, with no apparent reason, and you may lose your appetite. You may also find that your skin is itchy.

> **Obviously, most pain in the abdomen is not caused by cancer of the pancreas, but see your doctor if you are worried**

The rare islet cell tumours can sometimes cause symptoms by overproduction of insulin, which results in low levels of sugar in the blood. This may result in loss of energy and a feeling of weariness. It may also sometimes progress to attacks of dizziness and drowsiness.

The initial vague symptoms can be caused by many conditions other than cancer, but any persistent symptoms should always be discussed with your doctor to find out what has caused them.

# How does the doctor make the diagnosis?

Usually you begin by seeing your family doctor (general practitioner) who will examine you. As part of that examination he or she will look at your eyes and note the colour of your skin and will be able to detect any jaundice. He or she may also be able to feel a lump in your abdomen. After this examination your GP may arrange for you to have further tests or X-rays. He or she may need to refer you to hospital for these tests and for specialist advice and treatment. At the hospital the doctor will take your medical history before doing a physical examination. You may have a blood test and a chest X-ray to check your general health. The following tests are commonly used to diagnose cancer of the pancreas:

## *Ultrasound scan*

In this test sound waves are used to make up a picture of the area of the stomach and the liver. It will be done in the hospital scanning department. You should not eat or drink for at least 6 hours before the test.

Once you are lying comfortably on your back a gel is spread onto your abdomen. A small device, like a microphone, which produces sound waves, is then passed over the area. The echoes are converted into a picture using a computer. You will not hear these sounds.

Ultrasound can be used to measure the size and position of a cancer. It is a painless test and only takes a few minutes.

## *CT scan (CAT scan)*

In this scan several small X-rays are taken of the area in question and fed into a computer. This builds up a detailed picture of the size and position of the cancer.

Before the scan you will be asked to drink a special liquid which shows up on X-ray and ensures that a clear picture is obtained. Once you are lying in a comfortable position, the

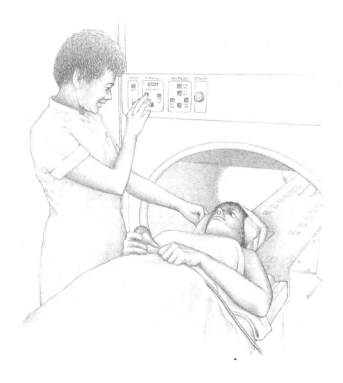

scan will be taken. The scan itself is painless but it will mean lying still for about 30-40 minutes.

You will probably be able to go home as soon as the scan is over.

### Magnetic resonance imaging (MRI or NMR scan)

This test is similar to a CT scan, but uses magnetism instead of X-rays to build up cross-sectional pictures of your body.

During the test you will be asked to lie very still on a couch inside a metal cylinder, which is open at both ends. The whole test may take up to an hour. It is completely painless, but lying inside the cylinder may make you feel claustrophobic. You can usually take someone with you into the room to keep you company.

It will probably take several days for the results of your tests to be ready and a follow-up appointment will be made for you. Obviously this waiting period is an anxious time. It will probably help if you can find a close friend or relative with whom to talk things over.

## ERCP (Endoscopic retrograde cholangio-pancreatography)

By using ERCP your doctor can obtain an X-ray picture of the pancreatic duct and the bile duct and can unblock the bile duct if needed (see page 17). You will be asked not to eat or drink anything for about six hours before the test so that the stomach and duodenum are empty. You will be given a tablet or injection to make you relax (a sedative). You may also be given an injection of antibiotics to prevent any infection. The doctor will then pass a thin, flexible tube known as an endoscope through your mouth, into your stomach and into the duodenum just beyond it. Looking down the endoscope the doctor can find the opening where the bile duct and the duct of the pancreas drain into the duodenum. A dye can be injected into these ducts which can be seen on X-ray and the doctor will be able to see if there are any abnormalities or any blockage of the duct.

Most people are able to go home the same day.

### Biopsy

The previous tests may make your doctor strongly suspect a diagnosis of cancer of the pancreas but the only certain way to make the diagnosis is to obtain some cells or a small piece of tissue to look at under a microscope. This can be obtained in a number of ways. Using ultrasound or a CT scan it may be possible to insert a fine needle through the skin of the abdomen and take a small piece of tissue. You will be given a local anaesthetic injection to ensure you feel no pain from the insertion of the needle. If the mass of the tumour is easily accessible, the doctor can use an automatic device to insert the needle into the tumour. A larger needle can be used with this method so a bigger sample of tissue can be obtained. The anaesthetic means you will feel no pain, but you might feel some slight discomfort as the needle is inserted.

Another way is to obtain some cells during ERCP (see previous page) when the doctor will be able to remove some fluid from the tumour through the endoscope. This is not, however, as satisfactory as obtaining a tissue sample.

If the doctor can't obtain a diagnosis by these means, a procedure called a laparotomy may be done under a general anaesthetic to obtain a piece of tissue. This involves making an incision in your abdomen so that the surgeon can take a sample of tissue from the pancreas.

# What types of treatment are used?

The type of treatment you are given will depend on a number of factors, including your age, your general health, the type of tumour you have, what it looks like under the microscope, the size of the cancer and how far it has spread, if at all. Treatment which is best for one person may not be right for someone else.

Surgery may be used to remove the cancer if it has not spread beyond the pancreas. It may also be used to treat a blockage of the bile duct or bowel if this occurs. Radiotherapy may be helpful in shrinking the cancer and for controlling pain. Chemotherapy may be used to treat cancers that have spread. Chemotherapy and radiotherapy may sometimes be given together, for cancers that cannot be removed by surgery but which have not spread beyond the pancreas.

You may find that other people at the hospital with cancer of the pancreas are having different treatment from you. This may be because their illness takes a different form and therefore they have different needs. It may also be because doctors take different views about treatment. If you have any questions about your own treatment, don't be afraid to ask your doctor or the nurse looking after you.

**It often helps to make a list of questions for your doctor and to take a close relative or friend with you**

Some people find it reassuring to have another medical opinion to help them decide about their treatment. Most doctors will be pleased to refer you to another specialist for a second opinion if you feel this will be helpful.

# Surgery

Occasionally it is possible to remove the entire cancer at an operation. This is a major operation, which is not suitable for everyone. If you are having surgery, you will need treatment beforehand to prepare you for it. Depending on where the cancer is situated and how much of the pancreas is involved, a part or all of the pancreas may need to be removed. During this operation a part of the stomach, duodenum, the common bile duct and the surrounding lymph nodes may also have to be removed.

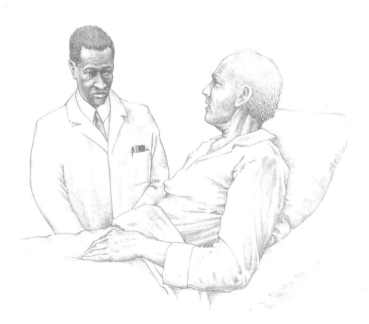

## After your operation

After your operation you may stay in an intensive care ward for the first couple of days. You will then be moved to a general ward until you recover. You will be encouraged to start moving about as soon as possible. This is an essential part of your recovery and even if you have to stay in bed it is important to keep up regular leg movements and deep breathing exercises. These will be explained to you by a physiotherapist.

An intravenous infusion (drip) will be used to replace your body's fluids until you are able to eat and drink again.

You may have a naso-gastric tube in place. This is a fine tube that passes down your nose into your stomach or small intestine and allows any fluids to be removed so that you don't feel sick. It is usually removed within 48 hours.

Often a small tube or catheter is put into your bladder and urine is drained into a collecting bag. This will save you having to get up to pass urine and is usually removed after a couple of days. You may also have a drainage tube in place from your wound to make sure that the wound heals properly.

After your operation you will probably have some pain and discomfort for a few days.

---

**There are several different types of very effective pain-killing drugs which you can take**

---

If you find that you are still in pain, let the nurses on the ward know as soon as possible so that your drugs can be reviewed.

You may also need to take capsules containing the enzymes which are normally produced by the pancreas. Some patients need to take insulin injections to regulate their blood sugar to replace the insulin normally produced by the pancreas.

## Bypass surgery

If the tumour blocks the bile duct, causing jaundice (see page 10), and it is not possible to remove it, then other procedures may be performed which relieve the blockage and allow the bile to go into the intestine. The jaundice will then clear up.

The surgical method of dealing with bile duct obstruction involves joining the gall bladder (or the bile duct) to part of your bowel (the jejunum). This bypasses the obstructed part of the bile duct by allowing the bile to flow from the liver into the intestine. This operation is called a cholecystojejunostomy if the gall bladder is used; choledochoenterostomy if the bile duct is used.

Another type of operation may be necessary to manage duodenal obstruction. This is called a gastrojejunostomy and involves connecting a piece of the bowel (the jejunum) to the stomach to bypass the duodenum. This will stop the persistent vomiting which can occasionally happen if the cancer blocks the duodenum.

## Jaundice

There are two ways in which it may be possible to relieve jaundice without a surgical operation; these methods are called endoscopic retrograde cholangiopancreatography (ERCP) and percutaneous transhepatic cholangiography (PTC).

The ERCP method involves the insertion of a tube, called a stent, to drain the bile which is building up in the duct. You will be asked not to eat or drink anything for six hours before the procedure so that the stomach and duodenum are empty. You will be given a sedative by injection, and the endoscope will be passed through your mouth as described on page 13. A dye will be used, as before. By looking at the X ray image the doctor will be able to see the narrowing in the bile duct. The narrowing can be stretched, using dilators, and a tube can be inserted through the endoscope, enabling the bile to drain. The tube usually needs to be replaced every three to four months to prevent it becoming blocked. There are few side effects from this procedure.

Another way of relieving the obstruction is the PTC method. This is similar to ERCP in that a dye is used to show up the obstruction on X-ray but instead of the plastic tube being inserted through an endoscope, a needle is inserted through your skin just below your rib cage and a guide is then passed through the obstruction in the bile duct into the duodenum. The plastic tube is then passed along this wire. As with ERCP, you will be asked not to eat or drink for at least six hours beforehand, and you will then be given a sedative. You will also have a local anaesthetic so you will not feel the needle or wire passing through your skin. Afterwards you may be given antibiotics to help prevent any infection. It is likely you will stay in hospital for a few days afterwards.

Sometimes, if the bile duct cannot be entered from the duodenum at ERCP, a combination of ERCP and PTC may be carried out.

# Radiotherapy

Radiotherapy may be used to treat cancer of the pancreas that cannot be removed by surgery, but which has not spread. It is often used together with chemotherapy (see page 21).

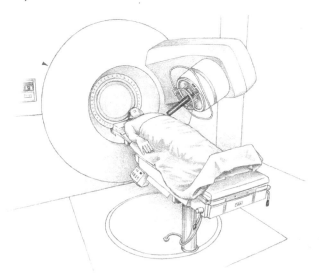

Radiotherapy is the use of high energy rays to destroy cancer cells, while doing as little harm as possible to normal cells.

Radiotherapy can be very helpful to relieve pain, and can also be used to try to shrink the cancer.

The treatment is given in the hospital radiotherapy department. The course is usually in five daily sessions from Monday to Friday, with a rest at the weekend, though some hospitals operate different regimes. The length of your treatment will depend on the type and size of the cancer. Your doctor will discuss your treatment with you in more detail beforehand.

## Planning your treatment

To ensure that you receive maximum benefit from your radiotherapy, it has to be carefully planned. On your first few visits to the radiotherapy department you will be asked to lie under a large machine called a simulator, which takes X-rays of the area to be treated. Sometimes a CT scanner can be used for the same purpose. Treatment planning is a very important part of radiotherapy and it may take a few visits before the radiotherapist, the doctor who plans and supervises your treatment, is satisfied with the result.

Marks may be drawn on your skin to help the radiographer, who gives you your treatment, to position you accurately and to show where the rays are to be directed. These marks must remain visible throughout your treatment but they can be washed off once your course is over. At the beginning of your radiotherapy you will be given instructions on how to look after the skin around the area being treated.

Before each session of radiotherapy the radiographer will position you carefully on the couch, either sitting or lying, and make sure you are comfortable. During your treatment, which only takes a few minutes, you will be left alone in the room, but you will be able to talk to the radiographer who will be watching you carefully from an adjoining room. Radiotherapy is not painful but you do have to be still for a few minutes while your treatment is being given.

## Side effects

Radiotherapy can cause general side effects such as nausea, vomiting, diarrhoea and tiredness. These side effects can be mild or more troublesome, depending on the strength of the radiotherapy dose and the length of your treatment. The radiotherapist will be able to advise you what to expect.

Nausea can usually be effectively treated by anti-sickness drugs (called anti-emetics), which your doctor can prescribe. If you don't feel like eating, you can replace meals with nutritious, high-calorie drinks which are available from most chemists and can be prescribed by your GP. BACUP's booklet *Diet and the cancer patient* has some helpful hints on how to eat well when you are feeling ill. Diarrhoea can be treated very effectively with drugs.

As radiotherapy can make you feel tired, try and get as much rest as you can, especially if you have to travel a long way for treatment each day.

All these side effects should disappear gradually once your course of treatment is over, but it is important to let your doctor know if they continue.

Radiotherapy does not make you radioactive and it is perfectly safe for you to be with other people, including children, throughout your treatment.

---

**BACUP publishes a booklet called**
***Understanding radiotherapy*, which gives**
**more details about this treatment**
**and its side effects**

---

# Chemotherapy

Chemotherapy is the use of special anti-cancer (cytotoxic) drugs to destroy cancer cells. The drugs work by disrupting the growth of cancer cells.

If the cancer is not operable, but has not spread beyond the pancreas, chemotherapy may be given together with radiotherapy to increase its effectiveness. If the cancer has spread, chemotherapy may be used to try and shrink the cancer and relieve symptoms. Any decision to use chemotherapy is usually reached after a discussion between you and your doctor.

Chemotherapy is usually given by injection into a vein (intravenously), either in your arm or via a plastic line called a central line in your chest. It is usually given as a course of treatment lasting a few days. This is followed by a rest period of a few weeks which allows your body to recover from any side effects of the treatment. The number of courses you have will depend on the type of cancer you have and how well it is responding to the drugs.

Chemotherapy may be given to you as an out-patient, but usually it will mean spending a few days in hospital.

## Side effects

Some drugs can cause side effects while others have none at all. Your doctor will tell you what problems, if any, to expect from your treatment.

While the drugs are acting on the cancer cells in your body, they also reduce temporarily the number of normal cells in your blood. When these cells are in short supply, you are more likely to get an infection and to tire easily. During chemotherapy your blood will be tested regularly and, if necessary, you will be given blood transfusions or antibiotics to treat any infection.

Some of the drugs used to treat cancer of the pancreas may cause nausea and vomiting. This can often be helped by taking anti-sickness drugs (anti-emetics) which your doctor can prescribe. Some chemotherapy drugs can make your mouth sore and cause small ulcers. Regular mouthwashes are important and the nurse will show you how to do these properly. If you don't feel like eating during treatment, you could try replacing some meals with nutritious drinks or a soft diet - BACUP's booklet *Diet and the cancer patient* has some useful tips on coping with eating problems.

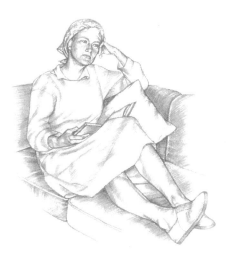

Unfortunately, hair loss is another common side effect of some - but not all - of these drugs. Ask your doctor if the drugs you are taking are likely to cause hair loss or other specific side effects. People who lose their hair often cover up by wearing wigs, hats or scarves. Most patients are entitled to a free wig from the National Health Service and your doctor or nurse will be able to arrange for a wig specialist to visit you. Although they may be hard to bear at the time, these side effects will disappear once your treatment is over, and if you lose your hair it will grow back surprisingly quickly. We would be pleased to send you a copy of BACUP's booklet, *Coping with hair loss*, if you think it would help you.

Chemotherapy affects people in different ways. Some find they are able to lead a fairly normal life during their treatment, but many find they become very tired and have to take things much more slowly. Just do as much as you feel like and try not to overdo it.

BACUP's booklet, *Understanding chemotherapy,* discusses the treatment and its side effects in more detail. Factsheets about individual drugs and their particular side effects are also available.

# Follow up

After your treatment has been completed your doctor will want you to have regular check-ups. These are a good opportunity to discuss with your doctor any worries or problems you may be having but if, in the meantime, you notice any new symptoms or are anxious about anything then contact your doctor or the ward sister for advice.

# Research – clinical trials

Research into new ways of treating cancer of the pancreas is going on all the time. Cancer doctors are continually looking for new ways to treat the disease and they do this by using clinical trials. Many hospitals now take part in these trials. BACUP holds a list of some current trials and can put you in touch with the appropriate organisation or doctor.

If early work suggests that a new treatment might be better than the standard treatment, cancer doctors will carry out trials to compare the new treatment with the best available standard ones. This is called a controlled clinical trial and is the only reliable way of testing a new treatment. Often several hospitals around the country take part in these trials.

So that the treatments can be compared accurately, the type of treatment a patient receives is decided at random - typically, by a computer - and not by the doctor treating the patient. This is because it has been shown that if a doctor chooses the treatment, or offers a choice to the patient, he or she may unintentionally bias the result of the trial.

In a randomised controlled clinical trial, some patients will receive the best standard treatment while others will receive the new treatment, which may or may not prove to be better than the standard treatment. A treatment is better either because it is more effective against the tumour or because it is equally effective and has fewer unpleasant side effects.

The reason why your doctor would like you to take part in a trial (or study as they are sometimes called) is because until the new treatment has been tested scientifically in this way it is impossible for doctors to know which is the best one to choose for their patients.

Before any trial is allowed to take place it must have been approved by an ethics committee. Your doctor must have your informed consent before entering you into any clinical trial. Informed consent means that you know what the trial is about, you understand why it is being conducted and why you have been invited to take part, and you appreciate exactly how you will be involved.

> **Even after agreeing to take part in a trial, you can still withdraw at any stage if you change your mind**

Your decision will in no way affect your doctor's attitude towards you. If you choose not to take part or you withdraw from a trial, you will then receive the best standard treatment rather than the new one with which it is being compared.

If you do choose to take part in a trial, it is important to remember that whatever treatment you receive will have been carefully researched in preliminary studies, before it is fully tested in any randomised controlled clinical trial.

By taking part in a trial you will also be helping to advance medical science and so improve prospects for patients in the future.

BACUP has a booklet called *Understanding clinical trials,* which explains clinical trials in more detail. We would be happy to send you a copy.

# Your feelings

Most people feel overwhelmed when they are told they have cancer. Many different emotions arise which can cause confusion and frequent changes of mood. You might not experience all the feelings discussed below or experience them in the same order. This does not mean, however, that you are not coping with your illness.

---

**Reactions differ from one person to another - there is no right or wrong way to feel**

---

These emotions are part of the process that many people go through in trying to come to terms with their illness. Partners, family members and friends often experience similar feelings and frequently need as much support and guidance in coping with their feelings as you do.

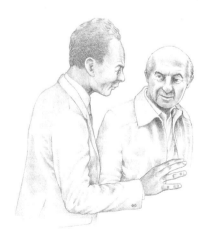

### Shock and disbelief

*'I can't believe it'; 'It can't be true'*

This is often the immediate reaction when cancer is diagnosed. You may feel numb, unable to believe what is happening or to express any emotion. You may find that you can take in only a small amount of information and so you have to keep asking the same questions over and over again, or you need to be told the same bits of information repeatedly. This need for repetition is a common reaction to shock. Some people may find their feelings of disbelief make it difficult for them to talk about their illness with their family and friends. Others may feel an overwhelming urge to discuss it with those around them. This may be a way of helping them to accept the news themselves.

BACUP has a booklet called *Who can ever understand? - talking about your cancer,* which we would be happy to send to you.

### Fear and uncertainty

*'Am I going to die?'; 'Will I be in pain?'*

Cancer is a frightening word surrounded by fears and myths. One of the greatest fears expressed by almost all newly diagnosed cancer patients is: 'Am I going to die?'

In fact, nowadays many cancers are curable if caught at an early enough stage. When a cancer is not completely curable, modern treatments often mean that the disease can be controlled for years and many patients can live an almost normal life.

Many people feel they need to sort out their affairs when they have been diagnosed with cancer, or any other potentially life-threatening illness. Doing so can take away some of that uncertainty, and reassure them that whatever happens their family will be looked after. One way to do this is to make a will, and BACUP has a booklet, *Will power,* which can help.

'Will I be in pain?' and 'Will any pain be unbearable?' are other common fears. In fact, many people with cancer feel no pain at all. For those who do, there are many modern drugs and other techniques which are very successful at relieving pain or keeping it under control. Other ways of easing pain or preventing you from feeling pain are radiotherapy and nerve blocks. BACUP has a booklet called *Feeling better - controlling pain and other symptoms of cancer* which may help you understand more about these procedures. We will be happy to send this to you.

Many people are anxious about their treatment - whether or not it will work and how to cope with possible side effects. It is best to discuss your individual treatment in detail with your doctor. Make a list of questions you may want to ask (see fill-in form at the end of this booklet).

---

### If you don't understand something about your treatment - ask

---

You may like to take a close friend or relative to the appointment with you. If you are feeling upset, they may be able to remember details of the consultation which you might have forgotten. You may want them to ask some of the questions you yourself might be hesitant of putting to the doctor.

Some people are afraid of the hospital itself. It can be a frightening place, especially if you have never been in one before, but talk about your fears to your doctor; he or she should be able to reassure you.

You may find the doctors can't answer your questions fully, or that their answers may sound vague. It is often impossible to say for certain that they have completely removed the tumour. Doctors know from past experience approximately how many people will benefit from a certain treatment, but it is impossible to predict the future for a particular person. Many people find this uncertainty hard to live with - not knowing whether or not you are cured can be disturbing.

Uncertainty about the future can cause a lot of tension, but fears are often worse than the reality. Gaining some knowledge about your illness can be reassuring. Discussing what you have found out with your family and friends can help to relieve tension caused by unnecessary worry.

## Denial

*'There's nothing really wrong with me'; 'I haven't got cancer'*

Many people cope with their illness by not wanting to know anything about it, or not wanting to talk about it. If that's the way you feel, then just say quite firmly to the people around you that you would prefer not to talk about your illness, at least for the time being.

Sometimes, however, it is the other way round. You may find that it is your family and friends who are denying your illness. They appear to ignore the fact that you have cancer, perhaps by playing down your anxieties and symptoms or deliberately changing the subject. If this upsets or hurts you because you want them to support you by sharing what you feel, try telling them. Start perhaps by reassuring them that you do know what is happening and that it will help you if you can talk to them about your illness.

## Anger

*'Why me of all people?'; 'And why right now?'*

Anger can hide other feelings such as fear or sadness and you may vent your anger on those who are closest to you and on the doctors and nurses who are caring for you. If you have a religious faith you may feel angry with your God.

It is understandable that you may be deeply upset by many aspects of your illness and there's no need to feel guilty about your angry thoughts or irritable moods. However, relatives and friends may not always realise that your anger is really directed at your illness and not against them. If you can, it may be helpful to tell them this at a time when you are not feeling quite so angry; or if you would find that difficult, perhaps you could show them this section of the booklet.

If you are finding it difficult to talk to your family, it may help to discuss the situation with a trained counsellor or psychologist. BACUP can give you details of how to get this sort of help in your area.

## Blame and guilt

*'If I hadn't ... this would never have happened'*

Sometimes people blame themselves or other people for their illness, trying to find reasons why it should have happened to them. This may be because we often feel better if we know why something has happened, but since doctors rarely know exactly what has caused an individual's cancer, there's no reason for you to blame yourself.

## Resentment

*'It's all right for you, you haven't got to put up with this'*

Understandably, you may be feeling resentful and miserable because you have cancer while other people are well. Similar feelings of resentment may crop up from time to time during the course of your illness and treatment for a variety of reasons. Relatives too can sometimes resent the changes that the patient's illness makes to their lives.

---

### Don't bottle up your feelings

---

It is usually helpful to bring these feelings out into the open so that they can be aired and discussed. Bottling up resentment can make everyone feel angry and guilty.

## Withdrawal and isolation

*'Please leave me alone'*

There may be times during your illness when you want to be left alone to sort out your thoughts and emotions. This can be hard for your family and friends who want to share this difficult time with you. It will make it easier for them to cope, however, if you reassure them that although you may not feel like discussing your illness at the moment, you will talk to them about it when you are ready.

Sometimes depression can stop you wanting to talk. It may be an idea to discuss this with your GP, who can prescribe a course of antidepressant drugs or refer you to a doctor or counsellor who specialises in the emotional problems of people with cancer.

## Learning to cope

After any treatment for cancer it can take a long time to come to terms with your emotions. Not only do you have to cope with the knowledge that you have cancer but also the physical effects of the treatment.

Although the treatment for cancer of the pancreas can cause unpleasant side effects, many people do manage to lead an almost normal life during their treatment. Obviously you will need to take time off for it, and some time afterwards to recover. Just do as much as you feel like and try to get plenty of rest.

---

**Everyone needs some support during difficult times**

---

It is not a sign of failure to ask for help or to feel unable to cope on your own. Once other people understand how you are feeling they can be more supportive.

# What to do if you are a friend or relative

Some families find it difficult to talk about cancer or share their feelings. It may seem best to pretend that everything is fine, and carry on as normal, perhaps because you don't want to worry the person with cancer or feel you are letting him or her down if you admit to being afraid. Unfortunately, denying strong emotions like this can make it even harder to talk, and lead to the person with cancer feeling very isolated.

Partners, relatives and friends can help by listening carefully to what and how much the person with cancer wants to say. Don't rush into talking about the illness. Often it is enough just to listen and let the person with cancer talk when she or he is ready.

BACUP has a booklet, *Lost for words*, written for relatives and friends of people with cancer. It looks at some of the difficulties people may have when talking about cancer, and suggests ways of overcoming them.

# Talking to children

Deciding what to tell your children about your cancer is difficult. How much you tell them will depend upon their age and how grown up they are. Very young children are concerned with immediate events. They usually need only simple explanations of why their relative or friend has had to go into hospital or isn't his or her normal self. Slightly older children may understand a story explanation in terms of good cells and bad cells. All children need to be repeatedly reassured that your illness is not their fault because, whether they show it or not, children often feel they may somehow be to blame and may feel guilty for a long time. Most children of about 10 years old and over can grasp fairly complicated explanations.

Adolescents may find it particularly difficult to cope with the situation because they feel they are being forced back into the family just as they were beginning to break free and gain their independence.

An open, honest approach is usually the best way for all children. Listen to their fears and be aware of any changes in their behaviour. This may be their way of expressing their feelings. It may be better to start by giving only small amounts of information and gradually building up a picture of your illness. Even very young children can sense when something is wrong, so don't keep them in the dark about what is going on. Their fears of what it might be are likely to be far worse than the reality.

---

**BACUP has a booklet called *What do I tell the children? - a guide for a parent with cancer,* which we would be happy to send you**

---

# What you can do

Many people feel helpless when they are first told they have cancer. They think there is nothing they can do, other than hand themselves over to doctors and hospitals. This is not so. There are many things you and your family can do at this time.

## Understanding your illness

If you and your family understand your illness and its treatment, you will be better prepared to cope with the situation. In this way you at least have some idea of what you are facing.

For information to be of value it must come from a reliable source to prevent it causing unnecessary fears. Personal medical information should come from your own doctor who is familiar with your medical background. As mentioned earlier, it can be useful to make a list of questions before your visit or take a friend or relative with you to remind you of things you want to know but can forget so easily. Other sources of information are given at the end of this booklet, along with a fill-in form to note your questions before you go to see the doctor or nurse.

## Practical and positive tasks

At times you may not be able to do things you used to take for granted. But as you begin to feel better you can set yourself some simple goals and gradually build up your confidence. Take things slowly and one step at a time.

Many people talk about 'fighting their illness'. This can help some people and you can do it by becoming involved in your illness. One easy way of doing this is by planning a healthy, well-balanced diet. Another way is to learn relaxation techniques which you can practise at home with audiotapes. BACUP has booklets called *Cancer and complementary therapies* and *Diet and the cancer patient*, which we would be happy to send to you.

Some people find that their experience of cancer has taught them to prioritise their time and use their energy more constructively than they did before their illness.

You may find it helpful to take some regular exercise. The type of exercise you take, and how strenuous, depends on what you are used to and how well you feel. Set yourself realistic aims and build up slowly.

If the idea of changing your diet or taking exercise does not appeal to you, then do not feel you have to do these things; just do whatever suits you. Some people may find pleasure in keeping to their normal routine as much as possible. Others prefer to take a holiday or spend more time on a hobby.

# Who can help?

The most important thing to remember is that there are people available to help you and your family. Often it is easier to talk to someone who is not directly involved with your illness. You may find it helpful to talk to a counsellor, who is specially trained to listen.

---

**BACUP's Cancer Counselling Service offers counselling at its London and Glasgow based offices**

---

The Counselling Service can tell you more about counselling and can let you know what services are available in your area (see page 37). Some people find great comfort in religion at this time and it may help for them to talk to a local minister, hospital chaplain or other religious leader.

There are several other people who can offer support in the community. District nurses work closely with GPs and make regular visits to some patients and their families at home. In many areas of the country there are also Macmillan and Marie Curie nurses, who are specially trained to look after people with cancer in their own homes. Let your GP know if you are having any problems so that proper home care can be arranged.

Some hospitals have their own emotional support services with specially trained staff, and some of the nurses on the ward will have been given training in counselling as well as being able to give advice about practical problems.

---

**You may qualify for benefits**

---

The hospital social worker is also often able to help in many ways such as giving information about social services and other benefits you may be able to claim while you are ill. For example, you may be entitled to meals on wheels, a home help or hospital fares. The social worker may also be able to help arrange childcare during and after treatment and, if necessary, help with the cost of childminders.

But there are people who require more than advice and support. They may find that the impact of cancer leads to depression, feelings of helplessness and anxiety. Specialist help in coping with these emotions is available in some hospitals. Ask your hospital consultant or GP to refer you to a doctor or counsellor who is an expert in the special emotional problems of cancer patients and their relatives.

## *Sick pay and benefits*

Incapacity Benefit has replaced Invalidity Benefit and Sickness Benefit. There are three rates of Incapacity Benefit: a short-term lower rate, a short-term higher rate, and a long-term rate.

If you are employed and unable to work, your employer can pay you Statutory Sick Pay (SSP) for a maximum of 28 weeks. If, after this period, you are still unable to work, you can claim the short-term higher rate of benefit from the Benefits Agency. After one year, if you are still unable to work, you can claim long-term Incapacity Benefit.

If you are self-employed, you are entitled to the same benefits as long as you have been paying the relevant Class 2 contributions.

People who are unemployed and unable to work will need to transfer from the Job Seekers Allowance to the short-term lower rate of Incapacity Benefit.

If you are ill and not at work, do remember to ask your family doctor for a medical certificate to cover the period of your illness. If you are in hospital, ask the doctor or nurse for a certificate, which you will need to claim benefit. You may also be required to take a medical test to assess whether or not you are eligible for benefit.

You may qualify for the Disability Living Allowance. Ask your family doctor for form DS1500.

The Benefits Agency has a form (IB202) which outlines all these benefits and others to which you may be entitled. You can get a copy from your local Citizens' Advice Bureau and Social Security office, who will also be able to advise you about the benefits you can claim. Their addresses and telephone numbers are in the phone book.

# BACUP's Cancer Support Service

## Information

Provides information on all aspects of cancer and its treatment, and on the practical and emotional problems of living with the illness. Information is on computer about services available to cancer patients, treatment and research centres, support groups, therapists, counsellors, financial assistance, insurance, mortgages and home nursing services. Some of these are listed on the following pages.

If you would like any other booklets, or help, you can phone and speak to one of our experienced cancer nurses. The service is open to telephone enquiries from 9am to 7pm Monday to Friday.

The number to call is: 0171 613 2121. You can call the information service free of charge on 0800 18 11 99.

## Counselling

Many people feel that counselling can help them deal with the problems of living with cancer. Counsellors use their skills to help people talk through the emotional difficulties linked to cancer. These are not always easy to talk about and are often hardest to share with those to whom you are closest. Talking with a trained counsellor who is not personally involved can help to untangle thoughts, feelings and ideas.

BACUP's cancer counsellors can give information about local counselling services and can discuss with people whether counselling could be appropriate and helpful for them. BACUP runs a one-to-one counselling service based at its London and Glasgow offices.

For more information about counselling or to make an appointment please ring 0171 696 9000 (London) or 0141 553 1553 (Glasgow).

# Useful organisations

**BACUP**
3 Bath Place
Rivington Street
London
EC2A 3JR
Office: 0171 696 9003

**BACUP Scotland**
**Cancer Counselling Service**
30 Bell Street
Glasgow
G1 1LG
Office: 0141 553 1553

**Information**
0171 613 2121 or Freephone: 0800 18 11 99
Open 9am-7pm Monday-Friday

**Counselling**
London:   0171 696 9000
Glasgow: 0141 553 1553

All BACUP's London numbers can take minicom calls.

Jersey BACUP
6 Royal Crescent, St Helier, Jersey JE2 4QG
Tel: 01534 89904 Freephone: 1200 275

*In addition to providing a link with BACUP's Cancer Information Service in the Channel Islands, Jersey BACUP runs a local cancer support group and trained local volunteers give support over the telephone, and in the local hospital.*

CancerLink
11-21 Northdown Street
London N1 9BN
Tel: 0171 833 2818
    0800 132905 (Freephone helpline)
    0800 590415 (Asian language helpline)

*Offers support and information on all aspects of cancer in response to telephone and letter enquiries. Acts as a resource to cancer support and self-help groups throughout the UK, and produces a range of publications on issues about cancer.*

Cancer Care Society
21 Zetland Road, Redland, Bristol BS6 7AH
Tel: 0117 942 7419/0117 923 2302

*Provides counselling and emotional support where possible through a network of support groups around the country. Holiday accommodation is available, and in some areas hospital visiting and help with transport.*

Macmillan Cancer Relief
Anchor House, 15-19 Britten Street, London SW3 3TZ
Tel: 0171 351 7811
(With regional offices throughout the country)

*Provides specialist advice and support through Macmillan nurses and doctors and financial grants for people with cancer and their families.*

Marie Curie Cancer Care
28 Belgrave Square, London SW1X 8QG
Tel: 0171 235 3325

*Runs eleven hospice centres for cancer patients throughout the UK, and a community nursing service which works in conjunction with the district nursing service to support cancer patients and their carers in their homes.*

Tak Tent Cancer Support – Scotland
Block C20, Western Court,
100 University Place, Glasgow G12 6SQ
Tel: 0141 211 1930/1/2

*Offers information, support, education and care for cancer patients, families, friends and professionals. Network of support groups throughout Scotland. 'Drop-in' Resource and Information Centre at the above address.*

Tenovus Cancer Information Centre
College Buildings, Courtenay Road, Splott, Cardiff CF1 1SA
Tel: 01222 497700
       0800 526527 (Freephone helpline)

*Provides an information service in English and Welsh on all aspects of cancer, and emotional support for cancer patients and their families. Operates a mobile screening unit, drop-in centre, support group and cancer helpline.*

The Ulster Cancer Foundation
40-42 Eglantine Avenue, Belfast BT9 6DX
Tel: 01232 663439 (helpline)
       01232 663281 (admin)

*Provides a cancer information helpline and resource centre, and support groups for patients and relatives. Produces a range of booklets.*


Hospice Information Service
St Christopher's Hospice, Lawrie Park Road, Sydenham, London SE26 6DZ
Tel: 0181 778 9252

*Provides a **Directory of Hospice Services** including in-patient units, home care support teams and hospital support teams in the UK and Eire.*

# Books recommended by BACUP

Robert Buckman
*What you really need to know about cancer: a comprehensive guide for patients and their families*
Macmillan, 1996
ISBN 0-333–61866-1   £20

Chapters on all types of cancer. Very comprehensive coverage, including sections on conventional and complementary treatments, screening, living with cancer and attitudes to cancer.

Nira Kfir and Maurice Slevin
*Challenging cancer: from chaos to control*
Tavistock/Routledge, 1991
ISBN 0-415-06344-2   £12.99

For people who have been diagnosed with cancer, their families and friends. Examines feelings and emotions with the help of a psychotherapist and a cancer doctor. Suggests ways people can regain control of their lives.

Val Speechley and Maxine Rosenfield
*Cancer information at your fingertips: the comprehensive cancer reference book for the 1990s* (2nd edn)
Class Publishing, 1996
ISBN 1-872362-56-7   £11.95

Questions and answers about cancer, its diagnosis, treatment, side effects, complementary therapies and life with cancer.

Hilary Thomas and Karol Sikora
*Cancer: a positive approach*
Thorsons, 1995
ISBN 0 7225-3132-X   £8.99

Information about all aspects of cancer and the treatments available. Also looks at the controversies in cancer, and includes checklists of questions to ask your doctor.

Jeffrey Tobias
*Cancer: what every patient needs to know*
Bloomsbury, 1995
ISBN 0-7475-1993-5   £6.99

Thorough and up-to-date coverage by a respected cancer
doctor.

Michael Whitehouse & Maurice Slevin
*Cancer: the facts*
Oxford University Press, 1996
ISBN 0-1926-1695-1   £8.99

Information on diagnosis and treatment of different types of
cancer. Also considers the emotional needs of cancer
patients, living with advanced cancer, and the role of
complementary medicine.

# BACUP booklets

## *Understanding cancer* series:

Acute lymphoblastic leukaemia
Acute myeloblastic leukaemia
Bladder
Bone cancer – primary
Bone cancer – secondary
Brain tumours
Breast – primary
Breast – secondary
Cervical smears
Cervix
Chronic lymphocytic leukaemia
Chronic myeloid leukaemia
Colon and rectum
Hodgkin's disease
Kaposi's sarcoma
Kidney
Larynx
Liver
Lung
Lymphoedema
Malignant melanoma
Mouth and throat
Myeloma
Non-Hodgkin's lymphoma
Oesophagus
Ovary
Pancreas
Prostate
Skin
Soft tissue sarcomas
Stomach
Testes
Thyroid
Uterus
Vulva

## *Understanding treatment* series:

Bone marrow and stem cell
   transplants
Breast reconstruction
Chemotherapy
Clinical trials
Radiotherapy
Tamoxifen factsheet

## *Living with cancer* series:

Complementary therapies
   and cancer
Coping at home: caring for
someone with advanced cancer
Coping with hair loss
Diet and the cancer patient
Facing the challenge of
   advanced cancer
Feeling better: controlling pain
   and other symptoms of cancer
Lost for words: how to talk to
   someone with cancer
Sexuality and cancer
What do I tell the children?
   – a guide for a parent with
   cancer
What now? Adjusting to life after
   cancer
Who can ever understand?
   – talking about your cancer
Will power – a step-by-step
   guide to making or changing
   your will

## Questions you might like to ask your doctor or surgeon

You can fill this in before you see the doctor or surgeon, and then use it to remind yourself of the questions you want to ask, and the answers you receive.

1. ...............................................................................................................

Answer ...................................................................................................

...............................................................................................................

2. ...............................................................................................................

Answer ...................................................................................................

...............................................................................................................

3. ...............................................................................................................

Answer ...................................................................................................

...............................................................................................................

4. ...............................................................................................................

Answer ...................................................................................................

...............................................................................................................

5. ...............................................................................................................

Answer ...................................................................................................

...............................................................................................................

6. ...............................................................................................................

Answer ...................................................................................................

...............................................................................................................